Natural Family Remedies
Cynthia Black

CONTENTS

Introduction

Before the days of supermarkets stocked with mounds of produce, shelves of manufactured cosmetics, and aisles of pharmeceutical drugs, it was important to know how to care for yourself and your household with common items from everyday life. Our families learned to use natural and herbal ingredients that were readily available and easy to apply for all sorts of purposes — among them beauty aids, health remedies, and household helpers. The recipes that my family created have been passed down through the generations. To this day, my family uses natural and herbal ingredients to create traditional remedies for all aspects of our everyday living. Your friends and family will appreciate these tried-and-true remedies that come from the heart and carry on traditions begun so long ago.

When you're working with herbs and other natural ingredients, it's important to pay close attention to the recipe instructions. More is not always better — 5 teaspoons of an herb in a hot-oil infusion will not necessarily work better than 2 teaspoons, and may in fact be harmful to your skin. Remember, the proportions called for in each recipe have been tested over time for best efficacy, so prepare the recipes as directed. In addition, use the recipes as directed — a remedy that is effective when applied externally may be toxic if taken internally.

Equipment

These recipes require only common utensils that can usually be found in your kitchen. Here's a list of the basic equipment you'll need:

- Stainless steel, enamel, or glass pot or saucepan
- Wooden spoon
- Double boiler
- Cheesecloth, colander, and/or press
- Nonmetal containers with lids
- Bottles of various sizes with caps

Definitions and Techniques

Before we begin, here are some definitions and instructions that will come in handy.

Creams. Herbal creams are easy to make. At your drugstore, buy a cream base that is hypoallergenic. Put this in the top of a double boiler and heat over boiling water, with the selected herbs, for 2 hours. (Unless otherwise directed, use about 1 ounce of dried herbs or 2½ ounces of fresh herbs per 10 ounces of cream base.) Remove from heat, strain through a cheesecloth, and pack into jars. Seal tightly and keep in a cool, dark place.

Decoctions. The term decoction refers to the method of extraction from tough plant material such as roots or bark. To make a decoction, combine herbs and cold water in a saucepan. (Unless otherwise directed, use about 1 ounce of dried herbs or 2 ounces of fresh herbs per 2 cups of water.) Bring to a boil and simmer gently for 20 to 40 minutes (or until the liquid is reduced by about one-third). Then strain the liquid into a container and cover. Store in a cool place or refrigerate. Decoctions are best when freshly made.

Infusions. Making infusions with fresh or dried herbs is similar to making tea — the herbs are steeped in liquid and then strained out. (Unless otherwise directed, use 1 tablespoon of fresh herbs or 2 teaspoons of dried herbs per cup of water.) To make a **cold infusion,** steep the herbs in cold water overnight in a sealed container. For a **hot infusion,** steep the herbs for 10 minutes in a covered container in hot water that has come down from a boil.

To make a **cold-oil infusion,** pack fresh herbs into a jar and add enough sunflower oil to cover them completely. Put a nonmetal lid on the jar (or a metal lid over a piece of plastic wrap stretched over the mouth of the jar) and place in the sun. Allow to steep for 3 to 4 weeks. Give the jar a gentle shake daily. Be sure that the herbs are completely immersed in the oil, or they can spoil. Strain and bottle. **For a hot-oil infusion,** combine fresh herbs and sunflower oil (or another unsaturated oil) in the top of a double boiler and heat over boiling water for 2 hours. (Unless otherwise directed, use 1 cup of fresh herbs per 2 cups of sunflower oil.) Do not allow the oil to boil. Strain the infused liquid through a piece of cheesecloth and store in bottles with tight-fitting lids in a cool, dark place.

Infused oils can be used for massage, bathing, cooking, or as the oil base of ointments.

Ointments. To make an ointment, melt unscented petroleum jelly in the top of a double boiler. Add the fresh herbs and cook for 3 hours. (Unless otherwise directed, use 1½ cups of fresh herbs per 2 cups of petroleum jelly.) Keep an eye on the bottom pot of water during this long cook, as it may boil dry. Remove from heat, strain, and pour into jars. Seal tightly and store in a cool, dark place. A shortcut in making an ointment, if you have some herbal infused oil, is merely to thicken it with some warmed beeswax.

Poultices. To make a poultice, place ground herbs inside a double layer of a cotton or muslin pad. Moisten with a small amount of water and apply externally. Use a tie of some sort to keep the poultice in place.

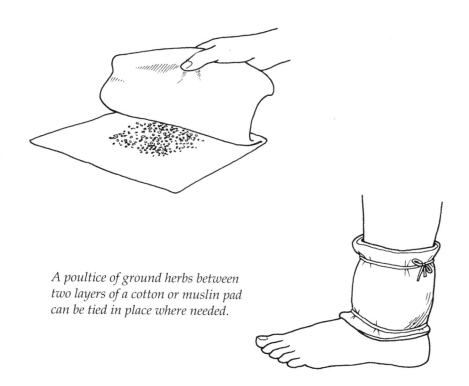

A poultice of ground herbs between two layers of a cotton or muslin pad can be tied in place where needed.

Tinctures. Tinctures are made by steeping herbs in a mixture of water and an alcohol such as vodka or gin (isopropyl alcohol, or rubbing alcohol, is extremely toxic — do not use in making tinctures). The alcohol/water mixture is usually in a ratio of 25 percent alcohol to 75 percent water, or 1 part alcohol to 3 parts water. This ratio must take into account the water already present in the alcohol; for example, if you use a bottle of vodka that contains only 37.5 percent alcohol, or roughly one-third, you will have to add water in the amount of one-third of the total volume of the vodka so that you have a final proportion of 3 parts water per 1 part alcohol in the final mixture.

Combine the herbs and alcohol/water mixture in a large container. (Unless otherwise directed, use 7 ounces of dried herbs or 21 ounces of fresh herbs per 4 cups of the water/alcohol mixture.) Be sure that the herbs are totally immersed in the liquid, or they may spoil. Cover and store in a cool place for 2 to 3 weeks, shaking occasionally. Then strain the mixture (for a more potent tincture, use a wine or cider press to press the herbs) and store in dark glass bottles. Tinctures will keep for up to two years.

Warning: Because of the alcohol content, tinctures should not be taken internally by pregnant or lactating women, children, or recovering alcoholics. Tinctures can be toxic if taken in excess; most remedies call for just 1 or 2 drops. Be sure to research the correct and safe dosage!

Recipes for Health and Healing

Natural and herbal healing has become a popular alternative to what we often consider traditional medicine — doctors, hospitals, and pharmaceutical drugs. Healing remedies that were once considered folklore have gained stature within the medical community as the natural healing properties of their ingredients are tested and approved. For further information about the growing use of herbs and natural ingredients for their healing properties, consult the great wealth of literature about homeopathy and natural healing.

Converting Recipe Measurements to Metric

Use the following formulas for converting U.S. measurements to metric. Since the conversions are not exact, it's important to convert the measurements for all of the ingredients to maintain the same proportions as the original recipe.

When The Measurement Given Is	Multiply It By	To Convert To
teaspoons	4.93	milliliters
tablespoons	14.79	milliliters
cups (liquid)	236.59	milliliters
cups (liquid)	0.236	liters
cups (dry)	275.31	milliliters
cups (dry)	0.275	liters
degrees Fahrenheit	fi/ª (temperature − 32)	degrees Celsius (Centigrade)

While standard metric measurements for dry ingredients are given as units of mass, U.S. measurements are given as units of volume. Therefore, the conversions listed above for dry ingredients are given in the metric equivalent of volume.

Skin Afflictions

Acne or broken skin: To soothe and smooth acne or broken skin, make a cold-oil infusion of plantain leaves and calendula petals (see instructions on page 3) and apply directly to your face with a moistened cotton ball.

Warts: To remove warts, rub them with fresh garlic or the white latex (sap) of dandelion stems.

Eczema: Make a cream using chickweed and violas (see instructions on page 3). Apply directly to the rash.

Insect bites I: Rub a minute amount of basil juice (which may be found at or ordered from a local natural foods store or herb shop) onto insect bites to help relieve itching.

Insect bites II: Make an ointment from 1 cup of fresh basil, ½ cup of fresh oregano, and 1 cup of fresh rosemary or fresh savory with 2 cups of petroleum jelly (see instructions on page 4). Spread over the bites. (Lesser quantities can be made by halving or quartering the recipe.)

Varicose veins and hemorrhoids: This astringent (for external use only) made from a decoction of witch hazel bark and leaves will shrink swollen tissue and ease varicose veins and hemorrhoids. Cut a branch of witch hazel into 2-inch pieces until you have ½ cup. Boil the pieces in 2 cups of water for 1 hour. Strain and add the resulting liquid to 1½ cups of water and 1½ cups of alcohol. Apply directly to your skin with a moistened cotton cloth, or fill a spray bottle and spritz it on. Store in the refrigerator for an extra cooling effect. You can also sprinkle some of this decoction in your bathwater.

Ringworm: This is an old remedy from my grandmother. Fill a small glass with vinegar, and then drop in 2 copper pennies. When the pennies are corroded and green, take them out and apply the vinegar to the ringworm.

Aches and Pains

Sore muscles I: Make a cold-oil infusion (see instructions on page 3) of sage and basil and massage into sore muscles.

Sore muscles II: A hot-oil infusion (see instructions on page 3) of comfrey and thyme will soothe aching muscles. Use 5 large comfrey leaves and 6 sprigs of thyme in 4 cups of oil. Heat in the top part of the double boiler for 3 hours.

Tense temples: Make a hot-oil infusion (see instructions on page 3) of 2 tablespoons of lavender and ½ cup of rose petals per 1½ cups of oil. Massage gently into tense temples.

Cuts and scrapes: For fast healing, mix a cream (see instructions on page 3) using calendula petals and apply directly to the affected area. Calendula cream is great to have in a first-aid kit.

Bruises and sprains I: I recently chipped my ankle bone in a fall. I made a poultice by grinding up 5 large comfrey leaves with 2 tablespoons of water in a blender and placed the mixture in a double layer of a cloth diaper. I put the poultice over my sore ankle and pulled a cotton sock over that foot to hold the poultice in place. The poultice stayed on all night. Although it did not relieve the pain, my ankle was barely bruised by the next day and healed very quickly.

Bruises and sprains II: Make a comfrey ointment (see instructions on page 4). Apply directly to the bruised or sprained area. Comfrey ointment can also be used to heal cuts.

Warning

Comfrey helps heal sprains and bruises externally, but it should never be taken internally; it may cause liver damage.

Raw or aching gums: Make a hot infusion (see instructions on page 3) using 1 cup of water and 1 teaspoon each of rosemary, sage, and mint. Allow the herbs to steep for 30 minutes before straining. Use as a mouthwash to ease sore gums.

Toothaches: My husband had a very sore tooth one evening, and as we live in a rural area, all the stores were closed. I remembered that my grandmother would rub clove oil on our gums when we had a toothache. Unfortunately, I did not have any clove oil for my husband, but I did have some cloves. He placed a clove on top of the molar that was bothering him, and although it did not totally eliminate the pain, the clove was warming and helped stop the intense throbbing. Although I do not recommend using cloves or clove oil in place of care from a dentist, it sure helped us until we could get to one.

Sore and inflamed feet: Use a small plastic tub or large pot to steep a couple of tablespoons of oregano in warm water. Soak your feet in the infused mixture.

Your Immune System

TINCTURE OF ECHINACEA

Echinacea is a powerful herb that helps stimulate the immune system. Use it only when you feel an illness coming on.

3   **good-size pieces of root of echinacea (purple coneflower)**

1   **cup vodka**

½   **cup boiled water, cooled**

Combine the root of echinacea and the vodka in a nonmetal container and cover. Allow to steep for 3 weeks. Strain liquid and mix with water. Store in a dark glass bottle in a cool place.

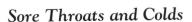

To use: Place 3 drops of this tincture on your tongue several times a day until you are feeling better.

Sore Throats and Colds

HOMEMADE PASTILLES

Pastilles (pronounced <u>pas-tee</u>) are throat soothers and can easily be made at home.

1½   **cups water**

1   **teaspoon dried horehound leaves**

⅛   **teaspoon dried thyme**

A pinch of dried mallow flower (if mallow is not available, you can use hollyhock or musk mallow)

2   **teaspoons dried mint leaves**

2¼   **cups sugar**

½   **teaspoon cream of tartar**

In a saucepan, bring the water to a boil and then remove from heat. Mix in the horehound, thyme, mallow flower, and mint and allow to steep for 1 hour. Strain into a separate pot. Add the sugar and cream of tartar to the strained liquid and stir over medium heat until the sugar is dissolved. Then cook without stirring until the mixture reaches the hard-crack stage (300°F). Pour into a greased pan. When it has cooled a bit, score into pieces. When completely hardened, break into smaller pieces.

For a lemon flavor, mix 1 teaspoon of dried horehound, a pinch of mallow, 2 tablespoons of fresh lemon balm, ½ teaspoon of lemon thyme, 2 teaspoons of dried mint, and a few drops of lemon oil. Proceed as directed above.

SYRUP TO SOOTHE THE THROAT

1½ cups water
1   tablespoon hyssop (the flowering tips of the plant are best)
½   teaspoon angelica
½   teaspoon mallow
1   cup rose hips
½   cup honey

In the top of a double boiler, combine the water, hyssop, angelica, mallow, and rose hips. Heat over boiling water for about 20 minutes, or until the hips are soft. Press through a colander and add honey to the strained liquid. Store in a covered container in the refrigerator.

GARGLES TO SOOTHE THE THROAT

Use this gargle when your throat is feeling scratchy.

½   teaspoon grated garlic or grated horseradish
¾   cup warm water
2   tablespoons honey

Mix the ingredients and gargle. Do not swallow!

For a simpler recipe, my grandmother added ½ teaspoon of salt to a glass of warm water and used this as a gargle.

TURNIP AND HONEY SYRUP
TO SOOTHE THE THROAT

Another old recipe for a scratchy throat is this old turnip-and-honey remedy.

1   medium-size rutabaga (also called a winter turnip)
Honey

Wash and peel the rutabaga. Slice it straight across the bottom to make it level so that it can sit up without falling over. Then cut the turnip into four equal wedges.

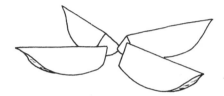

Slice the turnip across the bottom and then cut it into four equal wedges.

Spread the cut sides of each wedge with a liberal amount of honey and then put them back together again, re-forming your turnip. Set in a bowl to catch the juice. Cover the bowl and allow to sit for 24 hours, or until you see that you have collected a good amount of liquid in the bowl. Store the liquid in your refrigerator, and drink to soothe a scratchy throat.

OLD-FASHIONED MUSTARD PLASTER
FOR CHEST COUGHS

Here is an old remedy for chest coughs. Before penicillin and other antibiotics became widely available, pneumonia was a serious threat during the bitter winter months. My mother remembers using this mustard plaster during her yearly bouts with pneumonia.

¼   cup dry mustard
¼   cup flour
3   tablespoons molasses
Softened lard or thick cream

Mix the dry mustard with the flour and then stir in the molasses. Add enough softened lard or thick cream to make a workable ointment. Cover the sick person's throat and upper chest with a piece of flannel that has been dipped in warm water and wrung out. Apply

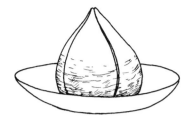

Re-form the turnip and set it in a bowl to catch the juice.

the mustard plaster to the throat and chest on top of the flannel cloth. Leave on for 15 minutes, or until the skin starts to redden.

Caution: This plaster can really heat up the skin, so monitor it carefully. Do not use if irritation develops.

CHEST RUBS FOR CHEST COLDS

These are two good chest rubs we use with good success.

Basil and Anise Chest Rub
- ½ cup basil
- ¼ cup anise or hyssop
- 2 cups oil

Mint and Thyme Chest Rub
- ½ cup mint
- ½ cup thyme
- 2 cups oil

Make a hot infusion using the herbs and oil. Massage into the chest area.

Warning: Do not use Basil and Anise Chest Rub during pregnancy. Potent applications of basil can have a stimulating effect on the uterus.

GARLIC

When you feel a cold coming on, chew up a clove of garlic twice a day. Garlic has many medicinal properties and is an antiseptic. We consider it a wonder plant. However, fresh garlic eaten alone can irritate the stomach if consumed in large quantities. To get around this, chop up a clove of garlic and sprinkle it on a nice green salad.

Healing Herbal Teas

In Europe, herbal teas are popularly called tisanes. This term comes from the Latin *ptisana*, which refers to a watery barley tea that was fed to the unwell. Today "tisane" can mean any healing or pleasurable tea of herbs. Tisanes are made as hot infusions. Boil your water and then remove from heat. Don't boil the tea once the herbs have been added! Pour the hot water over the herbs and cover. Let steep for 5 to 15 minutes, depending on how strong you want your tea to be. Strain and enjoy.

These are some recipes for teas that we have used for years. We try to use fresh ingredients. However, you can always substitute dried herbs for fresh — use 1 part of dried herbs in place of 2 parts of fresh herbs called for in the recipe.

FEMALE TEA

This tea serves as a wonderful relaxant during menstruation.

- 1   teaspoon fresh lemon basil
- 1   teaspoon fresh raspberry leaves
- 1½ cups water

HEADACHE TEA

This is a good remedy for a tension headache.

- 2   teaspoons fresh catnip
- 1½ cups water

RELAXING TEA

Chamomile is a well-known relaxant — drink this tea after a stressful day or as you're preparing for bed.

- 2   teaspoons fresh chamomile
- 1½ cups water

GASTROINTESTINAL RELIEF TEA

Fennel and anise will both work to relieve flatulence.

- 1   teaspoon fennel
- 1   teaspoon anise
- 1½ cups water

DIGESTIVE TEA

This tea will help ease digestion problems.

1   teaspoon fresh mint
1   teaspoon fresh bee balm
1½ cups water

CURE-ALL TEA

This is my all-time favorite tea. I've used it for just about every health problem.

1   tablespoon fresh lemon balm
1   tablespoon fresh mint
2   teaspoons chamomile
2   teaspoons chopped rose hips
2½ cups water

Recipes for Natural Beauty

If you want to care for yourself and your body naturally, look to herbs and other natural ingredients for some of the purest remedies available. These are recipes that my family has made and used through the generations.

Remedies for Skin Problems

Dry or rough skin: Add borage juice (which may be found at or ordered from a local natural foods store or herb shop) to skin creams to help soften your skin. You can also make a cream (see instructions on page 3) using calendula petals, chamomile flowers, rose petals, and elderberry flowers.

Toning face mask: Combine 2 tablespoons of oatmeal, 1 egg white (not beaten), and 1 tablespoon of honey to make a wonderful face mask that helps tone the skin. With your hands, mix these three ingredients in a small bowl and then apply the mixture directly to your face.

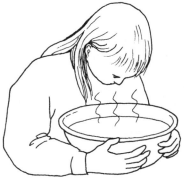

Facial cleanser: Apply buttermilk or yogurt to the face and leave it on for 15 to 20 minutes to help reduce large pores. For the same effect, you can also steep 1 tablespoon of fresh rosemary in a pot of very hot water and gently steam your face.

Oily skin: Mix ½ cup of apple juice and 2 teaspoons of witch hazel. Apply directly to your face with a moistened cotton ball (or put in a spray bottle and spritz on your face).

Wrinkles: Sage has long been known to help combat wrinkles. Make a cold infusion (see instructions on page 3) using 1 part sage per 2 parts water. Apply with a piece of very soft cotton (or put in a spray bottle and spritz).

Tired eyes: Place cucumber slices or spent black tea bags over your eyes to refresh them. Allow to stand for 5 to 10 minutes.

Stained hands: Remove stains with lemon juice (fresh or bottled) or vinegar.

Dry elbows: To soften dry elbows, rub them with a cold-oil infusion (see instructions on page 3) of calendula petals.

Callouses: To remove rough callouses, rub with salt.

Homemade Rose Water

You can make a cold infusion of rose petals to make homemade rose water, which is lovely applied to the face. Place 1 cup of chopped fresh rose petals in 2 cups of cold water and stir well. Let stand, covered, overnight and then strain. Use a cotton ball moistened with rose water to apply to your face, or fill a small spray bottle and spritz your face.

Herbal Soap

You can use a wide variety of herbs to make soaps from hot infusions. Consult an herbal reference, or check with a local herb shop, to find which herbs yield the qualities you desire, and then mix and match to find the combinations you like best. Herbal soaps make wonderful gifts: Wrap them in netting and tie with a festive bow.

BASIC SOAP RECIPE

⅓ cup boiling water
2 tablespoons chopped chamomile flowers
1 tablespoon calendula petals
½ teaspoon chopped sage
2 bars glycerin or unscented, nondeodorant soap, grated

Pour the boiling water over the chamomile flowers, calendula petals, and sage. Let steep overnight. Then, if you want a clear soap, strain the herbs from the hot-infused liquid. You can also opt to leave the herbs in the soap — mixing the herbs into the soap can create a wonderful decorative effect. Place the grated soap and the herbal infusion in the top of a double boiler. Heat over boiling water until well mixed. Let cool until you can handle the soap, and then form the mixture into small shapes such as ovals or balls. Place them on cookie sheets and allow to dry for 2 weeks.

For oily skin: Add 1 teaspoon of rosemary and 1 tablespoon of cornmeal to the herb mixture prior to the hot infusion.

Hair Care

Dandruff: Mix equal parts of vinegar and water and use as a final hair rinse. Leave in — there's no need to wash out the rinse.

Conditioning: Steep 1 teaspoon each of rosemary and chamomile in ¼ cup of hot water. Strain the infused liquid and add to it 1 tablespoon of vinegar and 1 beaten egg. Massage the mixture into freshly shampooed hair and let stand for 3 to 10 minutes. Rinse with lukewarm water.

Oily hair: To remove excess oil, sprinkle in some oatmeal or cornmeal and then brush it out.

Dry hair: Apply warm (not hot!) unsaturated oil to your hair. Cover with plastic, and then cover the plastic with a soft towel. Leave in for ½ hour to 2 hours, and then shampoo. You can also use herb-infused oil on your hair. Sage and rosemary are good choices for dark hair; chamomile for fair hair.

Hair rinse: Combine ½ cup of vinegar and 1 cup of water and bring to a boil. Remove from heat and add 2 tablespoons of rosemary and 1 tea bag (black tea for dark hair and chamomile for light). Let steep overnight, strain, and use the infused mixture as a final rinse.

Herbal Baths

Treat yourself to a relaxing herbal bath — one of the best cure-all remedies I know of. Add cold-infused herbal oil to your bathwater, or you can fill a cotton/muslin sachet or a recycled nylon stocking with dried or fresh herbs and let it steep like a giant tea bag in the bathwater. To soften bathwater, add ⅛ cup of baking soda.

Soothing bath: Combine fresh chamomile, calendula, rose petals, catnip, and witch hazel and steep in your bathwater. Or you can add a small amount of a cold-oil infusion of these herbs.

Skin-toning bath: Add ¼ cup of milk powder or ½ cup of milk to your bathwater to help soften your skin. (Cleopatra actually used to bathe in undiluted milk.) If your skin is oily, add ground oatmeal in a sachet.

Warning: These mixtures can make a slippery tub.

After-bath lotion: Make a cold infusion (see instructions on page 3) of rose petals and calendula flowers. Add 1 part rose petals to 2 parts water along with 1 tablespoon of calendula flowers per 1 cup of rose petals. Let steep overnight and strain. Apply with a piece of very soft cotton (or put in a spray bottle and spritz).

Footbath: Soak your tired or aching feet in 12 cups of warm water steeped with 1 tablespoon of comfrey, 2 teaspoons of mint, 2 teaspoons of rosemary, 2 teaspoons of calendula flowers, 1 teaspoon of thyme, and 1 teaspoon of sage, with 2 tablespoons of Epsom salts. You need not use all of these herbs at the same time — vary them until you come up with a favorite combination.

Recipes for Healthful and Healing Foods

Eating healthful and healing foods is an important part of caring for yourself. These traditional family recipes range from healing soups to eat when you are ill to healthful vegetable flours that you can use as a substitute in recipes that call for processed, bleached white flour. Adapt the recipes to suit your own palate, and enjoy!

Healing Soups

HERBAL BROTH

This herbal concoction is a wonderful source of nutrition during all types of illnesses. The warm steam of a hot soup soothes sore throats and lungs, and the clear liquid is easy to digest.

4	cups water
1	tablespoon fresh basil leaves
1	tablespoon fresh chervil leaves
1	tablespoon fresh parsley sprigs
1	tablespoon fresh spinach leaves
1	tablespoon fresh tarragon leaves
1	tablespoon fresh watercress leaves

In a medium-size saucepan, bring the water to a boil. Add the herbs, cover, and simmer for 10 minutes. Remove from heat and strain. Serve hot.

Herbal Humidifier

You can add fragrant moisture to a sickroom with an herbal mist. Make sure you do not use too much herb, or the fumes could be overpowering. I use about 1 tablespoon of basil and 2 teaspoons of thyme in 10 cups of water for the cool-mist humidifier.

VITAMIN SOUP

Our favorite vitamin-rich soup is great during the winter months. If you put your crockpot on low, you can simmer this soup almost all day. Try different combinations of herbs until you find your favorite tastes.

1	cup dried beans, any variety
⅓	cup dried peas
2	cups carrots, diced
2	cups potatoes, peeled and diced
2	cups parsnips, diced
1	cup rutabaga (turnip), diced
1	medium-size onion, chopped
2	teaspoons dried summer savory
½	teaspoon dried thyme
½	cup fresh or frozen parsley, chopped
2	cups cooked chicken (optional)
1	cup zucchini or pumpkin, grated (optional)

Soak the dried beans and peas in cold water for 8 hours (or overnight).

Fill the crockpot one-third full with water. Add the carrots, potatoes, parsnips, rutabaga, onion, beans, and peas. (If you decide to include them, add the cooked chicken and pumpkin or zucchini as well.) Let simmer for 3 hours, or until the vegetables are almost tender.

Add the summer savory, thyme, and parsley. Let simmer for another 1 to 2 minutes, or until vegetables are completely tender. Serve hot.

WHOLESOME BROTH

4	cups water
1	tablespoon sorrel, chopped
1	tablespoon lettuce, chopped
1	tablespoon chervil leaves, chopped
½	cup carrots, cut into matchsticks
¼	cup celery, cut into matchsticks
1	tablespoon green onion tops, chopped finely

In a medium-size saucepan, bring the water to a boil. Add the sorrel, lettuce, and chervil leaves and cook until tender (about 4 minutes). Remove from heat, cover, and let stand for 15 minutes.

Strain the mixture through a cheesecloth-lined colander. Return to heat, add the carrots and celery, and simmer until the vegetables are tender. Top with green onion, cook for 1 more minute, and then remove from heat. Serve hot.

VEGETABLE BOUILLON

This soup is delicious on its own, and also makes a great base for other dishes.

3	cloves garlic
4	medium-size onions
4	stalks celery
6	carrots
6	spinach leaves
4	tomatoes
2	tablespoons parsley
1	teaspoon thyme
2	teaspoons summer savory

Fill a large pot with water. Add all the ingredients and simmer until the vegetables are tender. Strain. (Our hens are more than happy to eat the resulting vegetable pulp.) If you wish, you can add some noodles or rice to the broth for a thick and delicious homemade soup. You can freeze the leftover vegetable bouillon.

Vinegar Tonics

CIDER TONIC

Cider tonic is a popular, healthful drink. It can ease indigestion and morning sickness, mitigate pain from arthritis and sinusitis, and reduce high blood alkalinity (which is often associated with chronic fatigue syndrome).

1	large glass water
1	teaspoon cider vinegar
1	teaspoon honey

Mix ingredients well and drink. You can substitute sparkling water or tonic for the water.

RASPBERRY SUMMER TONIC

This is an old family recipe that went down well after a hard day working on the farm.

½   cup sugar or honey
5   cups cider vinegar
3   cups fresh raspberries

Heat the sugar or honey in the vinegar until it is well dissolved. Remove from heat, let cool, and place in a large crock or glass jar. Add the fresh raspberries and cover. Make sure that the berries are totally covered. Allow to stand for 1 week, stirring or shaking gently each day. Then strain and bottle.

To use: Add 2 spoonfuls to 1 cup of water. Mix well and drink. More sugar or honey can be added if desired. You can substitute sparkling water or tonic for the water.

Healing with Yogurt

Yogurt has been used for centuries by physicians to help alleviate intestinal inflammations. You can also use yogurt as a substitute for cream cheese, cutting down on the fat and calories in your recipes.

YOGURT CHEESE

2   cups plain, no-fat (or low-fat) yogurt
Chives or other herbs of choice

Secure a cheesecloth across the top of a bowl. I lay a wooden spoon across the top of the bowl and then tie the corners of the cheesecloth around the middle of the spoon, so that the cloth hangs over the bowl like a pocket. Spoon the yogurt onto the cheesecloth and allow to drain overnight. The next day you should have yogurt cheese, the same consistency as cream cheese. Add herbs to taste (roughly 2½ tablespoons for me), mix well, and store in the refrigerator.

Homemade Fruit or Vegetable Flour

This healthful flour can be made from virtually any fruit or vegetable that has been dried. Slice and steam the vegetables, and then dry them in an oven set at its lowest temperature. Try substituting ½ cup of these flours for an equal amount of processed white flour in any recipe. Here are some guidelines for the flours we make.

Tomatoes: Slice the tomatoes about ¼ inch thick and steam for 2 minutes. Place the slices on cookie sheets and dry in your oven for 8 to 12 hours. When the slices are dry, grind them in a blender.

Carrots: Slice the carrots about ¼ inch thick and steam for 4 minutes. Place slices on cookie sheets and dry for 7 to 10 hours. Grind.

Spinach/chard/greens: Remove the stiff center rib from each leaf. Steam the leaves for 2 minutes. Place the leaves on cookie sheets and dry for 5 to 7 hours. Grind.

Sweet potatoes: Slice the sweet potatoes about ¼ inch thick and steam for 10 minutes. Place slices on cookie sheets and dry for 8 to 10 hours. Grind.

Apples: Peel, core, and slice the apples about ¼ inch thick. Steam the slices for 3 minutes. Dry the slices on cookie sheets in your oven for 6 to 10 hours. Grind.

Pears: Peel, core, and slice the pears about ¼ inch thick and steam for 2 minutes. Place the slices on cookie sheets and dry for 5 to 9 hours. Grind.

Recipes for Natural and Healing Scents

Aromas have been used in healing for centuries. Massage oils scented with fragrant herbs are very popular, as are herbal creams and lotions.

Simmer Pot Recipes

Simmer fragrant herbs and flowers in water (either in a pot on your stove burner, or in a container suspended above a candle) to fill a room with a range of scents. Replace the water in the simmer pot as necessary to keep it between one-quarter and one-half full. If you have a woodstove, you are indeed very lucky, as you can place your herbs and spices in a pot half filled with water and let it simmer all day.

Soothing scent: Lavender

Stimulating scent: Rosemary, sage, and basil

Refreshing scent: Use any combination of lemon balm, lemon thyme, lemon verbena, lemon mint, and lemon basil

Holiday scent: 2 pieces of 2-inch cinnamon bark, 8 cloves, ½ orange sliced in rounds, 1 tablespoon of pine needles

Aromatic Sachets

Before the advent of vacuum cleaners and washing machines, houses naturally contained many different aromas. Potpourri was often used in a variety of ways to help "freshen" the stale air of an enclosed area. To keep a room fresh, fragrant herbs were hidden under carpets and couch cushions. Lavender and scented geranium leaves were commonly used for this purpose, as well as sweet woodruff, which has a nice vanilla scent. You can still spread the wonderful aroma of potpourri: Gather the herbs together in a sachet and place them all over the house. Hang sachets in closets and bathrooms and tuck them under pillows or mattresses — just about anywhere you want them! You can make sachets from the traditional

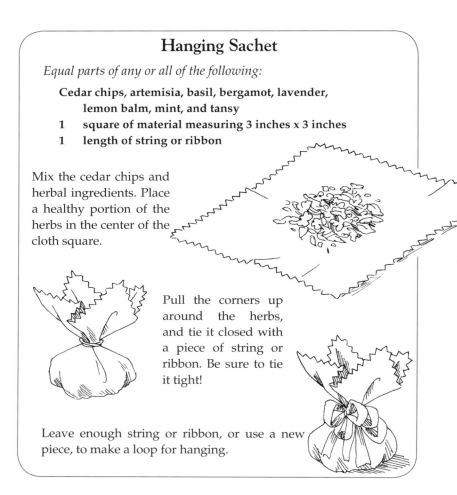

Hanging Sachet

Equal parts of any or all of the following:

> Cedar chips, artemisia, basil, bergamot, lavender,
> lemon balm, mint, and tansy
> 1 square of material measuring 3 inches x 3 inches
> 1 length of string or ribbon

Mix the cedar chips and herbal ingredients. Place a healthy portion of the herbs in the center of the cloth square.

Pull the corners up around the herbs, and tie it closed with a piece of string or ribbon. Be sure to tie it tight!

Leave enough string or ribbon, or use a new piece, to make a loop for hanging.

burlap or muslin that our great-grandparents had on hand (this material came from the bags used for holding oats and flour), or try a more decorative material. Sachets make great gifts!

SWEET NIGHTTIME SACHET

Sachets were often placed in pillows to sweeten the night air and induce relaxation.

> 2 parts hop vine flowers
> ½ part sweet woodruff flowers
> 1 part lady's mantle leaves and flowers

4	parts rose petals
½	part lavender
2	squares of material measuring 4 inches x 4 inches

Mix the herbal ingredients.

Sew together the squares of material by placing one on top of the other and stitching around the perimeter. Leave a 1-inch opening at one corner. Turn the sachet inside out and fill it with the herbal pot-pourri. Then stitch up the hole.

Place the sachet between your pillow and pillowcase.

You can avoid the sewing part altogether by using a piece of recycled nylon stocking as your sachet pocket. Stuff the stocking with the herbal potpourri. Make sure you tie the knot in the nylon tightly, or you'll end up with herbs everywhere!

Recipes for Home Care and Maintenance

This is a sampling of some traditional family recipes that we use to care for our household items. Be sure to use the proportions called for in the recipe, as too much or too little of any ingredient may render the recipe ineffective.

WOOD CONDITIONER

It's a good idea to first try this polish on a tiny spot on your furniture to determine if you like the effect.

2	tablespoons vinegar
1	tablespooon lemon or olive oil
1½	cups water

Mix together the ingredients. Warm the mixture slightly and apply to wood in minute amounts. Rub with a soft cloth.

FABRIC SOFTENER

2   teaspoons lavender
1   cup vinegar

Steep the lavender in the vinegar overnight in a nonmetal container or pot. Strain and add to the final rinse cycle of your wash.

WINDOW CLEANER

½   cup vinegar
6   cups warm water
Newspaper (no color sections)

Mix together the vinegar and warm water. Spray the mixture onto your windows and buff with a clean towel. Finish this procedure by buffing dried windows with newsprint.

TEAPOT CLEANER

2   cups vinegar
½   tablespoon baking soda
1   cup water

In the teapot, mix together the vinegar, baking soda, and water. Boil for 20 minutes and then rinse well.

Note: This recipe is for a large teapot. The mixture will foam up a bit in the pot.

Recipes for Mothers and Infants

Natural and herbal recipes make wonderful soothing and gentle remedies for mothers and babies. With infants, remember to test small amounts of any recipe before moving on to full-size doses or applications.

SITZ BATH

Comfrey has been traditionally used in sitz baths for perineal tears or soreness after childbirth.

2   cups comfrey leaves
4   cups water

Make a hot infusion (see instructions on page 3) of the comfrey leaves and water, allowing the herbs to steep for 1 hour. Strain.

Fill the tub with about 3 inches of water that is a bit warmer than usual, but not hot. Add 3 cups of the comfrey infusion. Sit in this bath, exposing the inflamed parts to the water as best you can. This will also soothe hemorrhoids.

DIAPER RASH OINTMENT

First check with your health care provider to diagnose any rash the baby may have. For a regular mild diaper rash, you can try this ointment. After application, let the baby go without a diaper for a while to let the air help heal the rash. When I first made this ointment, I tested it on the inside of my elbow for a week. When no irritation developed, I then tried a minute amount on my baby's bottom. Please do not use large amounts of any homemade ointment on your baby's skin until you are sure that it will not cause irritation.

2	cups unscented petroleum jelly
1	tablespoon chamomile flowers
1	tablespoon calendula flowers
½	cup plantain leaves
1	tablespoon lemon balm
2	teaspoons comfrey

Heat the herbs in the petroleum jelly in the top part of a double boiler for 3 hours. Then strain the mixture through a cotton cloth and store in jars. Apply sparingly to the irritated area.

RELAXING TEA FOR MOTHERS AND BABIES

Breast-feeding mothers can prepare this infusion, which always seems to settle nursing babies. I'm not really sure if this infusion calmed me and thus calmed the baby or if it calmed the baby via the breast milk!

2	teaspoons chamomile flowers
1	teaspoon fennel seeds
1	teaspoon catnip
2	cups heated water

Infuse the herbal ingredients in the heated water (see instructions on page 3). Drink the infusion as a tea with some honey.

ORGANIC BABY FOOD

Because we grow a huge organic garden, I never buy baby food. To make your own baby vegetable food, steam the vegetables (carrots, peas, and sweet potatoes are good beginner foods) and then puree them in the blender with a little of the cooking water. Spoon the mixture into ice-cube trays and place in the freezer. Once frozen (usually overnight), remove the vegetable cubes, put them in freezer bags, and store in the freezer. If the cubes are well sealed in bags and kept in a deep freeze, they should keep for 6 months to a year. Last year I found a bag of sweet dumpling squash cubes in the bottom of my freezer while I was spring cleaning. Since my baby was now eating solid foods, I used the cubes in our soups instead of throwing them in the compost.

Note: Introduce new vegetables one at a time. Try each one for a few days to make sure your baby is not allergic or sensitive to it.

Recipes for Animals

Traditional family remedies are not limited to the human members of our household — natural and herbal recipes are great for animals as well! You can use these recipes for the pets, livestock, and wild animals that are beloved members of your family.

HERBAL FLEA COLLARS

I use recycled nylon stockings to make flea collars and bed sachets for our cats and dog.

¼   cup cedar shavings
Pinch of dried garlic
1   teaspoon dried wormwood or artemisia
¼   teaspoon dried basil
1   tablespoon dried lemon balm
1   teaspoon dried mint or bergamot
A length of nylon stocking
Large handkerchief or bandanna

Mix together the cedar chips and herbal ingredients. Fill the nylon stocking with the mixture and tightly knot its end. Then place the stocking in the center of the handkerchief or bandanna, running diagonally so that the stocking ends are pointing to opposite corners.

Fold the hankie over the stocking, making a triangle, and roll it up beginning at the corner away from the stocking (the 90° angle corner). Roll into a narrow band and loosely tie around your pet's neck. Make sure that you do not tie the collar too tightly — and check the collar often to make sure that it does not tighten.

Note: If you are going to be away from your pet for a while, take the collar off until you return. Also, look for any signs of redness or irritation on your pet's skin underneath the collar. Although our animals have never developed any irritation, some animals have different sensitivities. If this irritation does occur, remove the collar.

You can also use this aromatic mixture to make sachets for your animals' sleeping quarters. Keep a sachet tucked under the bed or pad and out of chewing reach — wormwood and tansy can be toxic. Our dog sleeps in a large basket, and we place the sachets under the basket.

SKUNK DEODORIZER

Our dog recently had the misfortune of getting sprayed by a skunk. The skunk apparently took a fancy to our dog's prized bone, the dog retaliated by barking, and the upset skunk left behind a not-too-pleasant calling card. I got out some tomato juice, placed plastic bags over my hands, and rubbed the juice into the dog's coat. Luckily, it was summer and the dog's fur dried in about an hour. I brushed out the dried tomato residue and gave the dog a warm bath with ½ part vinegar mixed in 1 part water. The skunk smell was almost completely vanquished!

BARNYARD FLY REPELLENT

We keep a small flock of laying hens and ducks and always seem to have a problem with flies in the entryway of the barns. However, I find that the number of flies is significantly reduced when I hang up mixed bunches of tansy, basil, mint, bergamot, and catnip. You can also hang up 4-inch squares of yellow cardboard coated with tanglefoot.

HENHOUSE PORRIDGE

During the winter months I feel sorry for our hens, who must stay in the barn as temperatures plunge to around -40°F. I occasionally mix up a gruel hodgepodge to give them a treat in addition to their lay mash ration. All I do is boil up some potatoes, carrots, or other vegetables from the root cellar in some water. I add bran, fish waste, oatmeal, cornmeal, and some cracked wheat. If I have some leftover whey or skim milk, I also add that. Then I let the mixture cool before serving. This really perks the brood up, although it would be quite expensive to feed them this treat every day!

DOG BISCUITS

We call these tasty dog treats Canine Cookies.

1   cup unbleached flour
1   cup whole wheat flour
¾   cup cornmeal
½   cup wheat germ
1   cup beef bouillon
¼   cup Parmesan cheese
Pinch of garlic powder
2   eggs, beaten
½   cup finely chopped jerky or dried sausage (optional)

Preheat the oven to 300°F. Mix together all of the ingredients, adding a bit more flour if the mixture seems too sticky to handle. Roll out the dough about ½ inch thick. Cut into circles or other shapes and place on an ungreased cookie sheet. Bake for about 3 hours, or until the biscuits are rock hard. Turn off the heat and leave the biscuits in the oven overnight.

SUET CAKES

We feed the wild birds during the winter months. We usually grow an abundance of Mammoth sunflowers, which furnish a quantity of seed. What a delight to watch the evening grosbeaks, pine siskins, white-crowned sparrows, chickadees, chipping sparrows, cowbirds, jays, purple finches, goldfinches, and mourning doves. When -40°F hits, we supplement the seed with suet cakes, much enjoyed by nuthatches, woodpeckers, and flickers.

3   cups suet   1   cup peanut butter
Birdseed (sunflower seeds seem to be the most preferred).

Melt down the suet. Stir in the peanut butter, and let the mixture cool for about 5 minutes. Then stir in some birdseed. Pour the mixture into paper-lined muffin cups and let harden. Store it in the freezer to avoid rancidity. Remove the paper before setting the suet cakes in the bird feeders. Stop feeding suet when the coldest part of winter has passed, as it could interfere with the birds' breeding season and can be detrimental to their young.

Other Storey Titles You Will Enjoy

Natural BabyCare, by Colleen K. Dodt.
Pure and soothing herbal recipes and techniques
to promote the health of mothers and babies.
160 pages. Paper. ISBN-13: 978-0-88266-953-3.

Organic Body Care Recipes, by Stephanie Tourles.
Homemade, herbal formulas for glowing skin,
hair, and nails, plus a vibrant self.
384 pages. Paper. 978-1-58017-676-7.

***Rosemary Gladstar's Herbal Recipes
for Vibrant Health.***
A practical compendium of herbal lore and know-how
for wellness, longevity, and boundless energy.
408 pages. Paper. ISBN 978-1-60342-078-5.

***Rosemary Gladstar's Herbal Remedies
for Children's Health.***
How to use herbs such as chamomile, lemon balm,
and echinacea to create gentle baby care products
and safe treatments for childhood illnesses.
80 pages. Paper. ISBN 978-1-58017-153-3.

Rosemary Gladstar's Herbs for Natural Beauty.
An inspiring guide that offers a holistic approach to beauty
and includes the author's own Five-Step Skin Program.
80 pages. Paper. ISBN-13: 978-1-58017-152-6.

These and other books from Storey Publishing are available
wherever quality books are sold or by calling 1-800-441-5700.
Visit us at *www.storey.com*.